WE WANT TO BE PREGNANT

The ultimate guide on all you need to know about getting pregnant with IVF

Cassie Pierce

Table of Contents

CHAPTER 1

Overview of IVF

In vitro fertilization, also called IVF, is a complex series of procedures that can lead to a pregnancy. It's a treatment for infertility, a condition in which you can't get pregnant after at least a year of trying for most couples. IVF also can be used to prevent passing on genetic problems to a child.

Through IVF, eggs are manually fertilized using a sperm sample from a woman's partner or donor.

There are many ways to tailor the In Vitro Fertilization process to intended parents, from **reciprocal IVF** for lesbian couples, to **mini IVF treatments** for people searching for a lower-impact, less expensive approach to fertility.

IVF has helped many couples with fertility issues successfully conceive, and may be right for you if you have or experience:

- Damaged, blocked, or removed fallopian tubes
- Ovulation disorders, uterine fibroids, or premature ovarian failure
- Decreased sperm count or decreased sperm motility
- Unexplained infertility

Additionally, those who are in a same-sex relationships or are intended single parents can achieve their dream of building a family through IVF.

During in vitro fertilization, mature eggs are collected from ovaries and fertilized by sperm in a lab. Then a procedure is done to place one or more of the fertilized eggs, called embryos, in a uterus, which is where babies develop. One full cycle of IVF takes about 2 to 3 weeks. Sometimes these steps are split into different parts and the process can take longer.

In vitro fertilization is the most effective type of fertility treatment that involves the handling of eggs or embryos and sperm. Together, this group of treatments is called assisted reproductive technology.

IVF can be done using a couple's own eggs and sperm. Or it may involve eggs, sperm or embryos from a known or unknown donor. In some cases, a gestational carrier (someone who has an embryo implanted in the uterus) might be used.

Your chances of having a healthy baby using IVF depend on many factors, such as your age and the cause of infertility. What's more, IVF involves getting procedures that can be time-consuming, expensive and invasive. If more than one embryo is placed in the uterus, it can result in a pregnancy with more than one baby. This is called a multiple pregnancy.

CHAPTER 2

PREPARATION

To get started, you'll want to find a reputable fertility clinic.

A fertility clinic's success rate depends on many things. These include the ages and medical issues of people they treat, as well as the clinic's treatment approaches. When you talk with a representative at a clinic, also ask for detailed information about the costs of each step of the procedure.

Before you start a cycle of IVF using your eggs and sperm, you and your partner will likely need various screening tests. These include:

- Ovarian reserve testing. This involves getting blood tests to find out how many eggs are available in the body. This is also called egg supply. The results of the blood tests often used together with an ultrasound of the ovaries, can help predict how your ovaries will respond to fertility medicines.
- Semen analysis. Semen is the fluid that contains sperm. An analysis of it can check the amount of sperm, their shape, and how

they move. This testing may be part of an initial fertility evaluation. Or it might be done shortly before the start of an IVF treatment cycle.

- Infectious disease screening. You and your partner will both be screened for diseases such as HIV.
- Practice embryo transfer. This test doesn't place a real embryo in the uterus. It may be done to figure out the depth of your uterus. It also helps determine the technique that's most likely to work well when one or more actual embryos are inserted.
- Uterine exam. The inside lining of the uterus is checked before you start IVF. This might involve getting a test called sonohysterography. Fluid is sent through the cervix into the uterus using a thin plastic tube. The fluid helps make more detailed ultrasound images of the uterine lining. Or the uterine exam might include a test called hysteroscopy. A thin, flexible, lighted telescope is inserted through the vagina and cervix into the uterus to see inside it.

CHAPTER 3

TREATMENTS TO MAKE MATURE EGGS

The start of the IVF cycle begins by using lab-made hormones to help the ovaries to make eggs — rather than the single egg that usually develops each month. Multiple eggs are needed because some eggs won't fertilize or develop correctly after they're combined with sperm.

Certain medicines may be used to:

- Stimulate the ovaries. You might receive shots of hormones that help more than one egg develop at a time. The shot may contain a follicle-stimulating hormone (FSH), a luteinizing hormone (LH), or both.
- Help eggs mature. A hormone called human chorionic gonadotropin (HCG), or other medicines, can help the eggs ripen and get ready to be released from their sacs, called follicles, in the ovaries.
- Delay ovulation. These medicines prevent the body from releasing the developing eggs too soon.
- Prepare the lining of the uterus. You might start to take supplements of the hormone

progesterone on the day of the procedure to collect your eggs. Or you might take these supplements around the time an embryo is placed in the uterus. They improve the odds that a fertilized egg attaches to the lining of your uterus.

Your doctor decides which medicines to use and when to use them.

Most often, you'll need 1 to 2 weeks of ovarian stimulation before your eggs are ready to be collected with the egg retrieval procedure. To figure out when the eggs are ready, you may need:

- Vaginal ultrasound is an imaging exam of the ovaries to track the developing follicles. Those are the fluid-filled sacs in the ovaries where eggs mature.
- Blood tests, to check on how you respond to ovarian stimulation medicines. Estrogen levels often rise as follicles develop. Progesterone levels remain low until after ovulation.

Sometimes, IVF cycles need to be canceled before the eggs are collected. Reasons for this include:

- Not enough follicles develop.

- Ovulation happens too soon.
- Too many follicles develop, raising the risk of ovarian hyperstimulation syndrome.
- Other medical issues happen.

If your cycle is canceled, your care team might recommend changing medicines or the amounts you take, called doses. This might lead to a better response during future IVF cycles. Or you may be advised that you need an egg donor.

CHAPTER 4

EGG RETRIEVAL

This is the procedure to collect the eggs from one or both ovaries. It takes place in your doctor's office or a clinic. The procedure is done 34 to 36 hours after the final shot of fertility medicine and before ovulation.

- Before egg retrieval, you'll be given medicine to help you relax and keep you from feeling pain.
- An ultrasound device is placed into the vagina to find follicles. Those are the sacs in the ovaries that each contain an egg. Then a thin needle is inserted into an ultrasound guide to go through the vagina and into the follicles to collect the eggs. This process is called transvaginal ultrasound aspiration.
- If your ovaries can't be reached through the vagina this way, an ultrasound of the stomach area may be used to guide the needle through the stomach and into the ovaries.
- The eggs are removed from the follicles through a needle connected to a suction

device. Multiple eggs can be removed in about 20 minutes.
- After the procedure, you may have cramping and feelings of fullness or pressure.
- Mature eggs are placed in a liquid that helps them develop. Eggs that appear healthy and mature will be mixed with sperm to attempt to create embryos. However, not all eggs can be fertilized with success.

SPERM RETRIEVAL

If you're using your partner's sperm, a semen sample needs to be collected at your doctor's office or clinic on the morning of egg retrieval. Or sperm can be collected ahead of time and frozen.

Most often, the semen sample is collected through masturbation. Other methods can be used if a person can't ejaculate or has no sperm in the semen. For example, a procedure called testicular aspiration uses a needle or surgery to collect sperm directly from the testicle. Sperm from a donor also can be used. Sperms are separated from the semen fluid in the lab.

CHAPTER 5

FERTILIZATION

Two common methods can be used to try to fertilize eggs with sperm:

- Conventional insemination. Healthy sperm and mature eggs are mixed and kept in a controlled environment called an incubator.
- Intracytoplasmic sperm injection (ICSI). A single healthy sperm is injected right into each mature egg. Often, ICSI is used when semen quality or number is an issue. Or it might be used if fertilization attempts during prior IVF cycles didn't work.

In certain situations, other procedures may be recommended before embryos are placed in the uterus. These include:

- Assisted hatching. About 5 to 6 days after fertilization, an embryo "hatches" from the thin layer that surrounds it, called a membrane. This lets the embryo attach to the lining of the uterus. If you're older and you want to get pregnant, or if you have had past IVF attempts that didn't work, a technique called assisted hatching might be recommended. With this procedure, a hole is made in the embryo's membrane just before the embryo is placed in the uterus. This helps the embryo hatch and attach to the lining of the uterus. Assisted hatching is also useful for eggs or embryos that were frozen, as that process can harden the membrane.

- Preimplantation genetic testing. Embryos are allowed to develop in the incubator until they reach a stage where a small sample can be removed. The sample is tested for certain genetic diseases or the correct number of threadlike structures of DNA, called chromosomes. There are usually 46 chromosomes in each cell. Embryos that don't contain affected genes or chromosomes can be transferred to the uterus.
- Preimplantation genetic testing can lower the chances that a parent will pass on a genetic problem. It can't get rid of the risk completely. Prenatal testing may still be recommended during pregnancy.

CHAPTER 6

EMBRYO TRANSFER

The procedure to place one or more embryos in the uterus is done at your doctor's office or a clinic. It often takes place 2 to 6 days after eggs are collected.

- You might be given a mild sedative to help you relax. The procedure is often painless, but you might have mild cramping.
- A long, thin, flexible tube called a catheter is placed into the vagina, through the cervix and into the uterus.
- A syringe that contains one or more embryos in a small amount of fluid is attached to the end of the catheter.
- Using the syringe, the embryo or embryos are placed into the uterus.

If the procedure works, an embryo will attach to the lining of your uterus about 6 to 10 days after egg retrieval.

After the procedure

After the embryo transfer, you can get back to your usual daily routine. Your ovaries may still be enlarged, so vigorous activities or sex might cause discomfort. Ask your care team how long you should stay away from these.

Typical side effects include:

- Passing a small amount of clear or bloody fluid shortly after the procedure. This is due to the swabbing of the cervix before the embryo transfer.
- Breast tenderness due to high estrogen levels.
- Mild bloating.
- Mild cramping.
- Constipation.
- Fatigue.
- Headaches.
- Mood swing.
- Hot flashes.

When experiencing fatigue, cramping and other side effects, it's recommended you:

- Sleep for 8-10 hours every night
- Drink plenty of water
- Maintain a healthy, balanced diet
- Use approved over-the-counter pain relievers
- Rest warm compresses on areas of discomfort.

- Meditate and use other deep breathing or relaxation techniques.

Call your care team if you have moderate or severe pain or heavy bleeding from the vagina after the embryo transfer. You'll likely need to get checked for complications such as infection, twisting of an ovary, and ovarian hyperstimulation syndrome.

CHAPTER 7

RESULTS

At least 12 days after egg retrieval, you get a blood test to find out whether you're pregnant.

- If you're pregnant, you'll likely be referred to an obstetrician or other pregnancy specialist for prenatal care.
- If you're not pregnant, you'll stop taking progesterone and likely get your period within a week. Call your care team if you don't get your period or if you have unusual bleeding. If you'd like to try another cycle of IVF, your care team might suggest steps you can take to improve your chances of getting pregnant next time.

The chances of giving birth to a healthy baby after using IVF depend on various factors, including:

- Maternal age. The younger you are, the more likely you are to get pregnant and give birth to a healthy baby using your eggs during IVF. Often, people 40 and older are counseled to think about using donor eggs during IVF to boost their chances of success.

- Embryo status. Transfer of embryos that are more developed is linked with higher pregnancy rates compared with less-developed embryos. However, not all embryos survive the development process. Talk with your care team about your specific situation.
- Reproductive history. People who've given birth before are more likely to be able to get pregnant using IVF than are people who've never given birth. Success rates are lower for people who've already tried IVF multiple times but didn't get pregnant.
- Cause of infertility. Having an average supply of eggs raises your chances of being able to get pregnant using IVF. People who have severe endometriosis are less likely to be able to get pregnant using IVF than those who have infertility without a clear cause.
- Lifestyle factors. Smoking can lower the chance of success with IVF. Often, people who smoke have fewer eggs retrieved during IVF and may miscarry more often. Obesity also can lower the chances of getting pregnant and having a baby. The use of alcohol, drugs, too much caffeine, and certain medicines also can be harmful.

Talk with your care team about any factors that apply to you and how they may affect your chances of a successful pregnancy.

CHAPTER 8

RISKS

IVF raises the chances of certain health problems. From short term to longer term, these risks include:

- Stress. IVF can be draining for the body, mind, and finances. Support from counselors, family, and friends can help you and your partner through the ups and downs of infertility treatment.
- Complications from the procedure to retrieve eggs. After you take medicines to spur the growth of sacs in the ovaries that each contain an egg, a procedure is done to collect the eggs. This is called egg retrieval. Ultrasound images are used to guide a long, thin needle through the vagina and into the sacs, also called follicles, to harvest the eggs. The needle could cause bleeding, infection, or damage to the bowel, bladder, or blood vessels. Risks are also linked with medicines that can help you sleep and prevent pain during the procedure, called anesthesia.
- Ovarian hyperstimulation syndrome. This is a condition in which the ovaries become

swollen and painful. It can be caused by receiving shots of fertility medicines, such as human chorionic gonadotropin (HCG), to trigger ovulation. Symptoms often last up to a week. They include mild belly pain, bloating, upset stomach, vomiting and diarrhea. If you become pregnant, your symptoms might last a few weeks. Rarely, do some people get a worse form of ovarian hyperstimulation syndrome that also can cause rapid weight gain and shortness of breath.

- Miscarriage. The rate of miscarriage for people who conceive using IVF with fresh embryos is similar to that of people who conceive naturally — about 15% for pregnant people in their 20s to over 50% for those in their 40s. The rate rises with the pregnant person's age.
- Ectopic pregnancy. This is a condition in which a fertilized egg attaches to tissue outside the uterus, often in a fallopian tube. The embryo can't survive outside the uterus, and there's no way to continue the pregnancy. A small percentage of people who use IVF will have an ectopic pregnancy.
- Multiple pregnancy. IVF raises the risk of having more than one baby. Becoming

pregnant with multiple babies carries higher risks of pregnancy-related high blood pressure and diabetes, early labor and delivery, low birth weight, and birth defects than does pregnancy with a single baby.

- Birth defects. The age of the mother is the main risk factor for birth defects, no matter how the child is conceived. However assisted reproductive technologies such as IVF are linked with a slightly higher risk of a baby being born with heart issues, digestive problems, or other conditions. More research is needed to find out if it's IVF that causes this raised risk or something else.
- Premature delivery and low birth weight. Research suggests that IVF slightly raises the risk that the baby will be born early or with a low birth weight.
- Cancer. Some early studies suggested that certain medicines used to stimulate egg growth might be linked with getting a specific type of ovarian tumor. But more-recent studies do not support these findings. There doesn't seem to be a significantly higher risk of breast, endometrial, cervical, or ovarian cancer after IVF.